VETERINARY CONTROLLED SUBSTANCE LOG BOOK

NAME _____

ADDRESS _____

_____

_____

PHONE _____

EMAIL _____

LOG START DATE _____

LOG END DATE _____

LOG BOOK NUMBER _____

NOTES _____

_____

_____

Drug Name :				Strength :			

Date	Patient Name	Client ID	Initial Amount	Amount Removed	Amount Remains	Authorized By	Dispensed By

NOTE : _____
_____
_____
_____

Drug Name :					Strength :		
Date	Patient Name	Client ID	Initial Amount	Amount Removed	Amount Remains	Authorized By	Dispensed By

NOTE : _____
_____
_____
_____

Drug Name :					Strength :		

Date	Patient Name	Client ID	Initial Amount	Amount Removed	Amount Remains	Authorized By	Dispensed By

NOTE : _____
_____
_____
_____

Drug Name :   Strength :

Date	Patient Name	Client ID	Initial Amount	Amount Removed	Amount Remains	Authorized By	Dispensed By

NOTE : _____
_____
_____
_____

Drug Name :					Strength :		
Date	Patient Name	Client ID	Initial Amount	Amount Removed	Amount Remains	Authorized By	Dispensed By

NOTE : _____
_____
_____
_____

Drug Name :						Strength :	
Date	Patient Name	Client ID	Initial Amount	Amount Removed	Amount Remains	Authorized By	Dispensed By

NOTE : _____
_____
_____
_____

Drug Name :						Strength :	

Date	Patient Name	Client ID	Initial Amount	Amount Removed	Amount Remains	Authorized By	Dispensed By

NOTE : _____
_____
_____
_____

Drug Name :   Strength :

Date	Patient Name	Client ID	Initial Amount	Amount Removed	Amount Remains	Authorized By	Dispensed By

NOTE :

Drug Name :				Strength :			
Date	Patient Name	Client ID	Initial Amount	Amount Removed	Amount Remains	Authorized By	Dispensed By

NOTE : _____
_____
_____
_____

Drug Name :					Strength :		
Date	Patient Name	Client ID	Initial Amount	Amount Removed	Amount Remains	Authorized By	Dispensed By

NOTE : _____
_____
_____
_____

Drug Name :						Strength :	
Date	Patient Name	Client ID	Initial Amount	Amount Removed	Amount Remains	Authorized By	Dispensed By

NOTE : _____
_____
_____
_____

Drug Name :						Strength :	
Date	Patient Name	Client ID	Initial Amount	Amount Removed	Amount Remains	Authorized By	Dispensed By

NOTE : _____
_____
_____
_____

Drug Name :					Strength :		
Date	Patient Name	Client ID	Initial Amount	Amount Removed	Amount Remains	Authorized By	Dispensed By

NOTE : _____

_____

_____

_____

Drug Name :						Strength :	
Date	Patient Name	Client ID	Initial Amount	Amount Removed	Amount Remains	Authorized By	Dispensed By

NOTE : _____
_____
_____
_____

Drug Name :					Strength :		
Date	Patient Name	Client ID	Initial Amount	Amount Removed	Amount Remains	Authorized By	Dispensed By

NOTE : _____
_____
_____
_____

Drug Name :					Strength :		
Date	Patient Name	Client ID	Initial Amount	Amount Removed	Amount Remains	Authorized By	Dispensed By

NOTE : _____
_____
_____
_____

Drug Name :				Strength :			
Date	Patient Name	Client ID	Initial Amount	Amount Removed	Amount Remains	Authorized By	Dispensed By

NOTE : _____
_____
_____
_____

Drug Name :				Strength :			
Date	Patient Name	Client ID	Initial Amount	Amount Removed	Amount Remains	Authorized By	Dispensed By

NOTE : _____
_____
_____
_____

Drug Name :					Strength :		
Date	Patient Name	Client ID	Initial Amount	Amount Removed	Amount Remains	Authorized By	Dispensed By

NOTE : _____
_____
_____
_____

Drug Name :					Strength :		
Date	Patient Name	Client ID	Initial Amount	Amount Removed	Amount Remains	Authorized By	Dispensed By

NOTE : _____
_____
_____
_____

Drug Name :   Strength :

Date	Patient Name	Client ID	Initial Amount	Amount Removed	Amount Remains	Authorized By	Dispensed By

NOTE : _____
_____
_____
_____

Drug Name :					Strength :		
Date	Patient Name	Client ID	Initial Amount	Amount Removed	Amount Remains	Authorized By	Dispensed By

NOTE : _____
_____
_____
_____

Drug Name :				Strength :			
Date	Patient Name	Client ID	Initial Amount	Amount Removed	Amount Remains	Authorized By	Dispensed By

NOTE : _____
_____
_____
_____

Drug Name :					Strength :		
Date	Patient Name	Client ID	Initial Amount	Amount Removed	Amount Remains	Authorized By	Dispensed By

NOTE : _____
_____
_____
_____

Drug Name :					Strength :		
Date	Patient Name	Client ID	Initial Amount	Amount Removed	Amount Remains	Authorized By	Dispensed By

NOTE : _____
_____
_____
_____

Drug Name :						Strength :	

Date	Patient Name	Client ID	Initial Amount	Amount Removed	Amount Remains	Authorized By	Dispensed By

NOTE : _____
_____
_____
_____

Drug Name :				Strength :			

Date	Patient Name	Client ID	Initial Amount	Amount Removed	Amount Remains	Authorized By	Dispensed By

NOTE : _____
_____
_____
_____

Drug Name :					Strength :		
Date	Patient Name	Client ID	Initial Amount	Amount Removed	Amount Remains	Authorized By	Dispensed By

NOTE : _____
_____
_____
_____

Drug Name :					Strength :		
Date	Patient Name	Client ID	Initial Amount	Amount Removed	Amount Remains	Authorized By	Dispensed By

NOTE : _____
_____
_____
_____

Drug Name :   Strength :

Date	Patient Name	Client ID	Initial Amount	Amount Removed	Amount Remains	Authorized By	Dispensed By

NOTE : _____
_____
_____
_____

Drug Name :   Strength :

Date	Patient Name	Client ID	Initial Amount	Amount Removed	Amount Remains	Authorized By	Dispensed By

NOTE : _____
_____
_____
_____

Drug Name :   **Strength :**

Date	Patient Name	Client ID	Initial Amount	Amount Removed	Amount Remains	Authorized By	Dispensed By

NOTE : _____
_____
_____
_____

Drug Name :				Strength :			

Date	Patient Name	Client ID	Initial Amount	Amount Removed	Amount Remains	Authorized By	Dispensed By

NOTE : _____
_____
_____
_____

Drug Name :					Strength :		
Date	Patient Name	Client ID	Initial Amount	Amount Removed	Amount Remains	Authorized By	Dispensed By

NOTE : _____
_____
_____
_____

Drug Name :				Strength :			

Date	Patient Name	Client ID	Initial Amount	Amount Removed	Amount Remains	Authorized By	Dispensed By

NOTE : _____
_____
_____
_____

Drug Name :				Strength :			
Date	Patient Name	Client ID	Initial Amount	Amount Removed	Amount Remains	Authorized By	Dispensed By

NOTE : _____
_____
_____
_____

Drug Name :				Strength :			
Date	Patient Name	Client ID	Initial Amount	Amount Removed	Amount Remains	Authorized By	Dispensed By

NOTE : _____
_____
_____
_____

Drug Name :   Strength :

Date	Patient Name	Client ID	Initial Amount	Amount Removed	Amount Remains	Authorized By	Dispensed By

NOTE : _____
_____
_____
_____

Drug Name :						Strength :	

Date	Patient Name	Client ID	Initial Amount	Amount Removed	Amount Remains	Authorized By	Dispensed By

NOTE : _____
_____
_____
_____

Drug Name :				Strength :			

Date	Patient Name	Client ID	Initial Amount	Amount Removed	Amount Remains	Authorized By	Dispensed By

NOTE : _____

_____

_____

_____

Drug Name :						Strength :	
Date	Patient Name	Client ID	Initial Amount	Amount Removed	Amount Remains	Authorized By	Dispensed By

NOTE : _____
_____
_____
_____

Drug Name :				Strength :			

Date	Patient Name	Client ID	Initial Amount	Amount Removed	Amount Remains	Authorized By	Dispensed By

NOTE : _____
_____
_____
_____

Drug Name :					Strength :		
Date	Patient Name	Client ID	Initial Amount	Amount Removed	Amount Remains	Authorized By	Dispensed By

NOTE : _____

_____

_____

_____

Drug Name :   Strength :

Date	Patient Name	Client ID	Initial Amount	Amount Removed	Amount Remains	Authorized By	Dispensed By

NOTE : _____
_____
_____
_____

Drug Name :					Strength :		
Date	Patient Name	Client ID	Initial Amount	Amount Removed	Amount Remains	Authorized By	Dispensed By

NOTE : _____
_____
_____
_____

Drug Name :				Strength :			
Date	Patient Name	Client ID	Initial Amount	Amount Removed	Amount Remains	Authorized By	Dispensed By

NOTE : _____
_____
_____
_____

Drug Name :					Strength :		
Date	Patient Name	Client ID	Initial Amount	Amount Removed	Amount Remains	Authorized By	Dispensed By

NOTE : _____
_____
_____
_____

Date	Patient Name	Client ID	Initial Amount	Amount Removed	Amount Remains	Authorized By	Dispensed By

Drug Name :   Strength :

NOTE :

Drug Name :						Strength :	
Date	Patient Name	Client ID	Initial Amount	Amount Removed	Amount Remains	Authorized By	Dispensed By

NOTE : _____
_____
_____
_____

Drug Name :				Strength :			
Date	Patient Name	Client ID	Initial Amount	Amount Removed	Amount Remains	Authorized By	Dispensed By

NOTE : _____
_____
_____
_____

Drug Name :						Strength :	
Date	Patient Name	Client ID	Initial Amount	Amount Removed	Amount Remains	Authorized By	Dispensed By

NOTE : _____
_____
_____
_____

Date	Patient Name	Client ID	Initial Amount	Amount Removed	Amount Remains	Authorized By	Dispensed By

Drug Name :   Strength :

NOTE : _____
_____
_____
_____

Drug Name :					Strength :		
Date	Patient Name	Client ID	Initial Amount	Amount Removed	Amount Remains	Authorized By	Dispensed By

NOTE : _____
_____
_____
_____

Drug Name :				Strength :			

Date	Patient Name	Client ID	Initial Amount	Amount Removed	Amount Remains	Authorized By	Dispensed By

NOTE : _____
_____
_____
_____

Drug Name :				Strength :			

Date	Patient Name	Client ID	Initial Amount	Amount Removed	Amount Remains	Authorized By	Dispensed By

NOTE : _____
_____
_____
_____

Drug Name :					Strength :		
Date	Patient Name	Client ID	Initial Amount	Amount Removed	Amount Remains	Authorized By	Dispensed By

NOTE : _____
_____
_____
_____

Drug Name :					Strength :		
Date	Patient Name	Client ID	Initial Amount	Amount Removed	Amount Remains	Authorized By	Dispensed By

NOTE : _____
_____
_____
_____

Drug Name :				Strength :			

Date	Patient Name	Client ID	Initial Amount	Amount Removed	Amount Remains	Authorized By	Dispensed By

NOTE : _____
_____
_____
_____

Drug Name :					Strength :		
Date	Patient Name	Client ID	Initial Amount	Amount Removed	Amount Remains	Authorized By	Dispensed By

NOTE : _____
_____
_____
_____

Drug Name :				Strength :			

Date	Patient Name	Client ID	Initial Amount	Amount Removed	Amount Remains	Authorized By	Dispensed By

NOTE : _____
_____
_____
_____

Drug Name :					Strength :		
Date	Patient Name	Client ID	Initial Amount	Amount Removed	Amount Remains	Authorized By	Dispensed By

NOTE : _____
_____
_____
_____

Date	Patient Name	Client ID	Initial Amount	Amount Removed	Amount Remains	Authorized By	Dispensed By

Drug Name :   Strength :

NOTE :

Drug Name :					Strength :		
Date	Patient Name	Client ID	Initial Amount	Amount Removed	Amount Remains	Authorized By	Dispensed By

NOTE : _____
_____
_____
_____

Drug Name :					Strength :		

Date	Patient Name	Client ID	Initial Amount	Amount Removed	Amount Remains	Authorized By	Dispensed By

NOTE : _____
_____
_____
_____

Drug Name :						Strength :	
Date	Patient Name	Client ID	Initial Amount	Amount Removed	Amount Remains	Authorized By	Dispensed By

NOTE : _____
_____
_____
_____

Drug Name :					Strength :		

Date	Patient Name	Client ID	Initial Amount	Amount Removed	Amount Remains	Authorized By	Dispensed By

NOTE : _____

_____

_____

_____

Drug Name :					Strength :		
Date	Patient Name	Client ID	Initial Amount	Amount Removed	Amount Remains	Authorized By	Dispensed By

NOTE : _____
_____
_____
_____

Date	Patient Name	Client ID	Initial Amount	Amount Removed	Amount Remains	Authorized By	Dispensed By

Drug Name :　　　　　　　　　　　　Strength :

NOTE :　_____
　　　　　_____
　　　　　_____
　　　　　_____

Drug Name :				Strength :			

Date	Patient Name	Client ID	Initial Amount	Amount Removed	Amount Remains	Authorized By	Dispensed By

NOTE : _____
_____
_____
_____

Drug Name :				Strength :			

Date	Patient Name	Client ID	Initial Amount	Amount Removed	Amount Remains	Authorized By	Dispensed By

NOTE : _____
_____
_____
_____

Drug Name :					Strength :		
Date	Patient Name	Client ID	Initial Amount	Amount Removed	Amount Remains	Authorized By	Dispensed By

NOTE : _____
_____
_____
_____

Date	Patient Name	Client ID	Initial Amount	Amount Removed	Amount Remains	Authorized By	Dispensed By

Drug Name :   Strength :

NOTE : _____
_____
_____
_____

Date	Patient Name	Client ID	Initial Amount	Amount Removed	Amount Remains	Authorized By	Dispensed By

Drug Name :   Strength :

NOTE : _____
_____
_____
_____

Drug Name :					Strength :		

Date	Patient Name	Client ID	Initial Amount	Amount Removed	Amount Remains	Authorized By	Dispensed By

NOTE : _____

_____

_____

_____

Drug Name :					Strength :		
Date	Patient Name	Client ID	Initial Amount	Amount Removed	Amount Remains	Authorized By	Dispensed By

NOTE : _____
_____
_____
_____

Drug Name :				Strength :			

Date	Patient Name	Client ID	Initial Amount	Amount Removed	Amount Remains	Authorized By	Dispensed By

NOTE : _____
_____
_____
_____

Drug Name :					Strength :		
Date	Patient Name	Client ID	Initial Amount	Amount Removed	Amount Remains	Authorized By	Dispensed By

NOTE : _____
_____
_____
_____

Drug Name :					Strength :		
Date	Patient Name	Client ID	Initial Amount	Amount Removed	Amount Remains	Authorized By	Dispensed By

NOTE : _____
_____
_____
_____

Drug Name :						Strength :	
Date	Patient Name	Client ID	Initial Amount	Amount Removed	Amount Remains	Authorized By	Dispensed By

NOTE : _____
_____
_____
_____

Drug Name :					Strength :		
Date	Patient Name	Client ID	Initial Amount	Amount Removed	Amount Remains	Authorized By	Dispensed By

NOTE : _____
_____
_____
_____

Drug Name :					Strength :		
Date	Patient Name	Client ID	Initial Amount	Amount Removed	Amount Remains	Authorized By	Dispensed By

NOTE : _____
_____
_____
_____

Drug Name :						Strength :	
Date	Patient Name	Client ID	Initial Amount	Amount Removed	Amount Remains	Authorized By	Dispensed By

NOTE : _____
_____
_____
_____

Drug Name :						Strength :	
Date	Patient Name	Client ID	Initial Amount	Amount Removed	Amount Remains	Authorized By	Dispensed By

NOTE : _____
_____
_____
_____

Drug Name :						Strength :	

Date	Patient Name	Client ID	Initial Amount	Amount Removed	Amount Remains	Authorized By	Dispensed By

NOTE : _____
_____
_____
_____

Drug Name :					Strength :		
Date	Patient Name	Client ID	Initial Amount	Amount Removed	Amount Remains	Authorized By	Dispensed By

NOTE : _____
_____
_____
_____

Drug Name :				Strength :			
Date	Patient Name	Client ID	Initial Amount	Amount Removed	Amount Remains	Authorized By	Dispensed By

NOTE : _____
_____
_____
_____

Drug Name :					Strength :		
Date	Patient Name	Client ID	Initial Amount	Amount Removed	Amount Remains	Authorized By	Dispensed By

NOTE : _____
_____
_____
_____

Drug Name :					Strength :			
Date	Patient Name	Client ID	Initial Amount	Amount Removed	Amount Remains	Authorized By	Dispensed By

NOTE : _____
_____
_____
_____

Drug Name :				Strength :			
Date	Patient Name	Client ID	Initial Amount	Amount Removed	Amount Remains	Authorized By	Dispensed By

NOTE : _____
_____
_____
_____

Drug Name :   Strength :

Date	Patient Name	Client ID	Initial Amount	Amount Removed	Amount Remains	Authorized By	Dispensed By

NOTE : _____
_____
_____
_____

Drug Name :						Strength :	
Date	Patient Name	Client ID	Initial Amount	Amount Removed	Amount Remains	Authorized By	Dispensed By

NOTE : _____

_____

_____

_____

Drug Name :   Strength :

Date	Patient Name	Client ID	Initial Amount	Amount Removed	Amount Remains	Authorized By	Dispensed By

NOTE : _____
_____
_____
_____

Drug Name :					Strength :		
Date	Patient Name	Client ID	Initial Amount	Amount Removed	Amount Remains	Authorized By	Dispensed By

NOTE : _____
_____
_____
_____

Date	Patient Name	Client ID	Initial Amount	Amount Removed	Amount Remains	Authorized By	Dispensed By

Drug Name :　　　　　　　　　　Strength :

NOTE :

Drug Name :				Strength :			

Date	Patient Name	Client ID	Initial Amount	Amount Removed	Amount Remains	Authorized By	Dispensed By

NOTE : _____
_____
_____
_____

Drug Name :					Strength :		
Date	Patient Name	Client ID	Initial Amount	Amount Removed	Amount Remains	Authorized By	Dispensed By

NOTE : _____
_____
_____
_____

Drug Name :				Strength :			
Date	Patient Name	Client ID	Initial Amount	Amount Removed	Amount Remains	Authorized By	Dispensed By

NOTE : _____
_____
_____
_____

Date	Patient Name	Client ID	Initial Amount	Amount Removed	Amount Remains	Authorized By	Dispensed By
Drug Name :						Strength :	

NOTE : _____
_____
_____
_____

Drug Name :					Strength :		
Date	Patient Name	Client ID	Initial Amount	Amount Removed	Amount Remains	Authorized By	Dispensed By

NOTE : _____
_____
_____
_____

Drug Name :   Strength :

Date	Patient Name	Client ID	Initial Amount	Amount Removed	Amount Remains	Authorized By	Dispensed By

NOTE : _____
_____
_____
_____

Date	Patient Name	Client ID	Initial Amount	Amount Removed	Amount Remains	Authorized By	Dispensed By

Drug Name :   Strength :

NOTE : _____
_____
_____
_____

Drug Name :   Strength :

Date	Patient Name	Client ID	Initial Amount	Amount Removed	Amount Remains	Authorized By	Dispensed By

NOTE : _____
_____
_____
_____

Drug Name :					Strength :		
Date	Patient Name	Client ID	Initial Amount	Amount Removed	Amount Remains	Authorized By	Dispensed By

NOTE : _____
_____
_____
_____

Date	Patient Name	Client ID	Initial Amount	Amount Removed	Amount Remains	Authorized By	Dispensed By

Drug Name : **Strength :**

NOTE : _____
_____
_____
_____

Drug Name :					Strength :		
Date	Patient Name	Client ID	Initial Amount	Amount Removed	Amount Remains	Authorized By	Dispensed By

NOTE : _____
_____
_____
_____

Drug Name :					Strength :		

Date	Patient Name	Client ID	Initial Amount	Amount Removed	Amount Remains	Authorized By	Dispensed By

NOTE : _____
_____
_____
_____

Drug Name :						Strength :	
Date	Patient Name	Client ID	Initial Amount	Amount Removed	Amount Remains	Authorized By	Dispensed By

NOTE : _____
_____
_____
_____

Drug Name :					Strength :		
Date	Patient Name	Client ID	Initial Amount	Amount Removed	Amount Remains	Authorized By	Dispensed By

NOTE : _____
_____
_____
_____

Drug Name :				Strength :			
Date	Patient Name	Client ID	Initial Amount	Amount Removed	Amount Remains	Authorized By	Dispensed By

NOTE : _____
_____
_____
_____

Date	Patient Name	Client ID	Initial Amount	Amount Removed	Amount Remains	Authorized By	Dispensed By

Drug Name :   Strength :

NOTE :

Drug Name :						Strength :	
Date	Patient Name	Client ID	Initial Amount	Amount Removed	Amount Remains	Authorized By	Dispensed By

NOTE : _____
_____
_____
_____

Drug Name :					Strength :			
Date	Patient Name	Client ID	Initial Amount	Amount Removed	Amount Remains	Authorized By	Dispensed By

NOTE : _____
_____
_____
_____

Drug Name :					Strength :		
Date	Patient Name	Client ID	Initial Amount	Amount Removed	Amount Remains	Authorized By	Dispensed By

NOTE : _____
_____
_____
_____

Drug Name :				Strength :			

Date	Patient Name	Client ID	Initial Amount	Amount Removed	Amount Remains	Authorized By	Dispensed By

NOTE : _____

_____

_____

_____

Drug Name :						Strength :	
Date	Patient Name	Client ID	Initial Amount	Amount Removed	Amount Remains	Authorized By	Dispensed By

NOTE : _____
_____
_____
_____

Drug Name :				Strength :			
Date	Patient Name	Client ID	Initial Amount	Amount Removed	Amount Remains	Authorized By	Dispensed By

NOTE : _____
_____
_____
_____

Drug Name :					Strength :		
Date	Patient Name	Client ID	Initial Amount	Amount Removed	Amount Remains	Authorized By	Dispensed By

NOTE : _____
_____
_____
_____

Date	Patient Name	Client ID	Initial Amount	Amount Removed	Amount Remains	Authorized By	Dispensed By

Drug Name :   Strength :

NOTE : _____
_____
_____
_____

Drug Name :					Strength :		
Date	Patient Name	Client ID	Initial Amount	Amount Removed	Amount Remains	Authorized By	Dispensed By

NOTE : _____
_____
_____
_____

Made in the USA
Monee, IL
23 December 2021

87018958R00070